The Vibrant Vegetarian Cookbook

Easy And Delicious Vegetarian Recipes For Everyone

Adam Denton

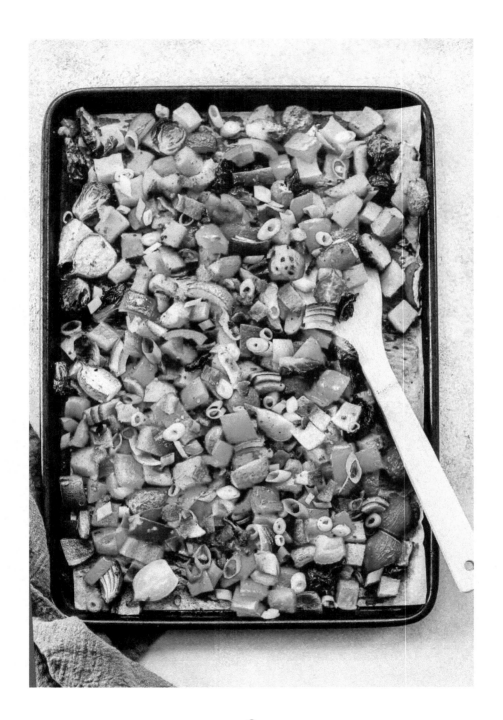

Table of contents

5

Jalapeno Kale and Parsnips

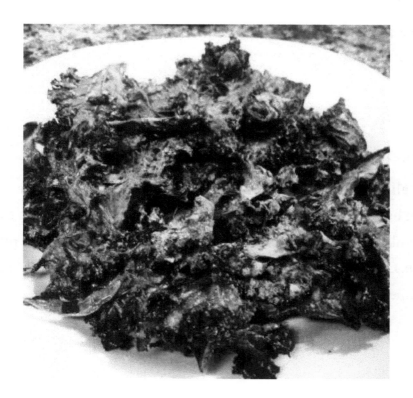

Ingredients

1 ½ pounds parsnips, peeled and cut into 1-inch chunks

½ red onion, thinly sliced

¼ cup water

½ vegetable stock cube, crumbled

1 tbsp. extra virgin olive oil

½ tsp cumin

½ tsp jalapeno pepper, minced

1 ancho chili, minced

Black pepper

½ pound Kale, roughly chopped

Directions:

Put all of the Ingredients in a slow cooker except the last one. Top with handfuls of kale and stuff the slow cooker with it. If you can't fit it all in at once, let the first batch cook first and add some more Kale. Cook for 3or 4 hours on medium until parsnips become soft. Scrape the sides and serve.

Spicy Choy Sum and Broccoli

Ingredients

1 pound broccoli, peeled and cut into 1-inch chunks

½ pound button mushrooms, sliced

½ onion, thinly sliced

¼ cup water

½ vegetable stock cube, crumbled

1 tbsp. sesame oil

½ tsp Chinese five spice powder

½ tsp Sichuan peppercorns

½ tsp hot chili powder

Black pepper

½ pound choy sum, roughly chopped

Directions:

Put all of the Ingredients in a slow cooker except the last one. Top with handfuls of choy sum and stuff the slow cooker with it. If you can't fit it all in at once, let the first batch cook first and add some more choy sum. Cook for 3or 4 hours on medium until broccoli become soft. Scrape the sides and serve.

Kale and Potatoes in Pesto Sauce

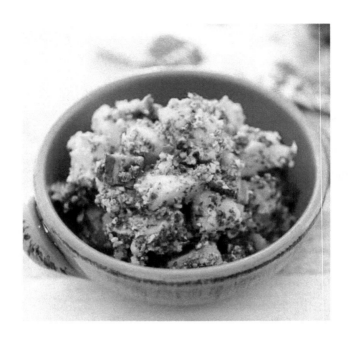

Ingredients

1 ½ pounds potatoes, peeled and cut into 1-inch chunks

½ onion, thinly sliced

¼ cup vegetable stock

1 tbsp. extra virgin olive oil

2 tbsp. pesto sauce

Black pepper

½ pound fresh Kale, roughly chopped

Directions:

Put all of the Ingredients in a slow cooker except the last one. Top with handfuls of Kale and stuff the slow cooker with it. If you can't fit it all in at once, let the first batch cook first and add some more Kale. Cook for 3 or 4 hours on medium until potatoes become soft. Scrape the sides and serve.

Turnip Greens and Kohlrabi in Pesto Sauce

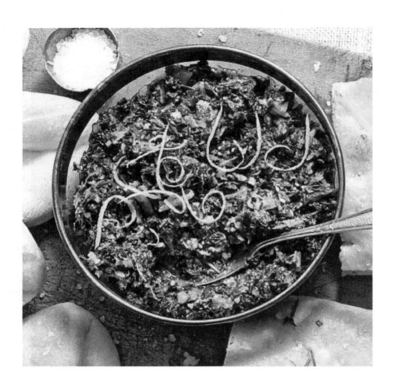

Ingredients

1 ½ pounds kohlrabi,peeled and cut into 1-inch chunks

½ onion, thinly sliced

¼ cup vegetable stock

1 tbsp. extra virgin olive oil

2 tbsp. pesto sauce

Black pepper

½ pound fresh Turnip Greens, roughly chopped

Directions:

Put all of the Ingredients in a slow cooker except the last one. Top with handfuls of Turnip Greens and stuff the slow cooker with it. If you can't fit it all in at once, let the first batch cook first and add some more Turnip Greens. Cook for 3or 4 hours on medium until kohlrabi become soft. Scrape the sides and serve.

Bok Choy and Kohlrabi in Chili Garlic Sauce

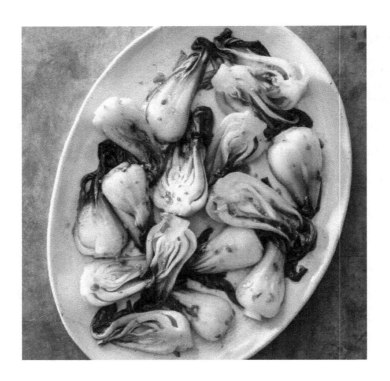

Ingredients

1 ½ pounds kohlrabi, peeled and cut into 1-inch chunks

½ onion, thinly sliced

¼ cup vegetable stock

1 tbsp. sesame oil

4 cloves garlic, minced

2 tbsp. chili garlic sauce

Black pepper

½ pound fresh Bok Choy, roughly chopped

Directions:

Put all of the Ingredients in a slow cooker except the last one. Top with handfuls of Bok Choy and stuff the slow cooker with it. If you can't fit it all in at once, let the first batch cook first and add some more Bok Choy. Cook for 3 or 4 hours on medium until kohlrabi become soft. Scrape the sides and serve.

Slow Cooked Kale and Summer Squash

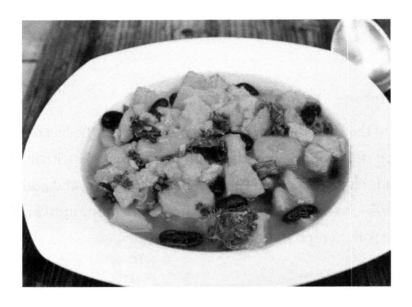

Ingredients

1 ½ pounds summer squash, peeled and cut into 1-inch chunks

½ onion, thinly sliced

¼ cup vegetable stock

1 tbsp. extra virgin olive oil

2 tbsp. pesto sauce

Black pepper

½ pound fresh Kale, roughly chopped

Directions:

Put all of the Ingredients in a slow cooker except the last one. Top with handfuls of kale and stuff the slow cooker with it. If you can't fit it all in at once, let the first batch cook first and add some more kale. Cook for 3or 4 hours on medium until summer squash become soft. Scrape the sides and serve.

Slow-cooked Endives and Brussel Sprouts

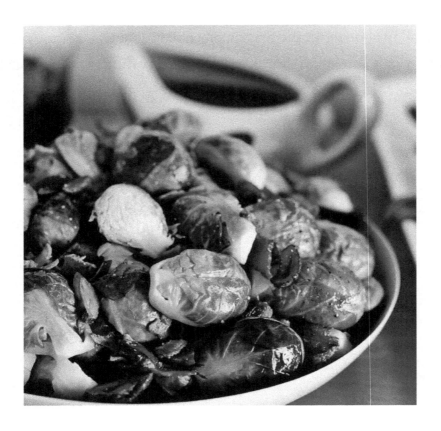

Ingredients

1 ½ pounds brussel sprouts

½ onion, thinly sliced

¼ cup vegetable stock

1 tbsp. extra virgin olive oil

Black pepper

½ pound fresh endives, roughly chopped

Directions:

Put all of the Ingredients in a slow cooker except the last one. Top with handfuls of endives and stuff the slow cooker with it. If you can't fit it all in at once, let the first batch cook first and add some more endives. Cook for 3 hours on medium until brussel sprouts become soft. Scrape the sides and serve.

Buttery Swiss Chard and Turnips

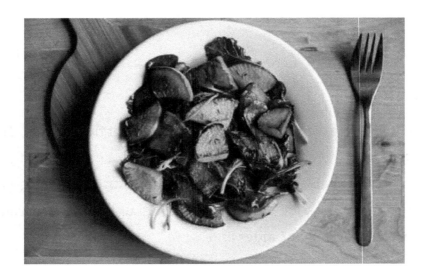

Ingredients

1 ½ pounds turnips, peeled and cut into 1-inch chunks

½ onion, thinly sliced

¼ cup vegetable stock

4 tbsp. vegan butter or margarine

2 tbsp. lime juice

3 cloves garlic, minced

Black pepper

½ pound fresh swiss chard, roughly chopped

Directions:

Put all of the Ingredients in a slow cooker except the last one. Top with handfuls of swiss chard and stuff the slow cooker with it. If you can't fit it all in at once, let the first batch cook first and add some more swiss chard. Cook for 3or 4 hours on medium until turnips become soft. Scrape the sides and serve.

Slow Cooked Chinese Style Choy Sum & Carrots

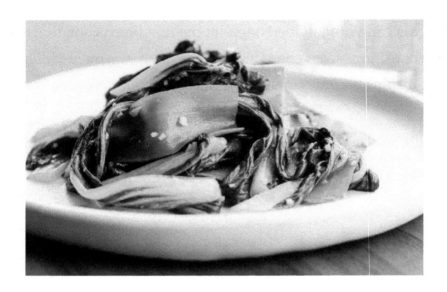

Ingredients

1 ½ pounds carrots, peeled and cut into 1-inch chunks

½ onion, thinly sliced

¼ cup vegetable stock

1 tbsp. sesame oil

2 tbsp. hoi sin sauce

Black pepper

½ pound choy sum, roughly chopped

Directions:

Put all of the Ingredients in a slow cooker except the last one. Top with handfuls of choy sum and stuff the slow cooker with it. If you can't fit it all in at once, let the first batch cook first and add some more choy sum. Cook for 3or 4 hours on medium until carrots become soft. Scrape the sides and serve.

Slow Cooked Micro greens and Potatoes

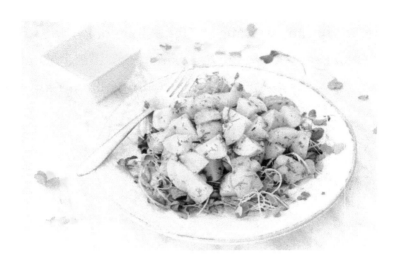

Ingredients

1 ½ pounds potatoes, peeled and cut into 1-inch chunks

½ onion, thinly sliced

¼ cup vegetable stock

2 tbsp. extra virgin olive oil

1 tsp. annatto seeds

1 tsp. cumin

1 tsp. lime juice

Black pepper

½ pound fresh Micro greens, roughly chopped

Directions:

Put all of the Ingredients in a slow cooker except the last one. Top with handfuls of micro greens and stuff the slow cooker with it. If you can't fit it all in at once, let the first batch cook first and add some more micro greens. Cook for 3or 4 hours on medium until potatoes become soft. Scrape the sides and serve.

Slow Cooked Red Cabbage and Potatoes

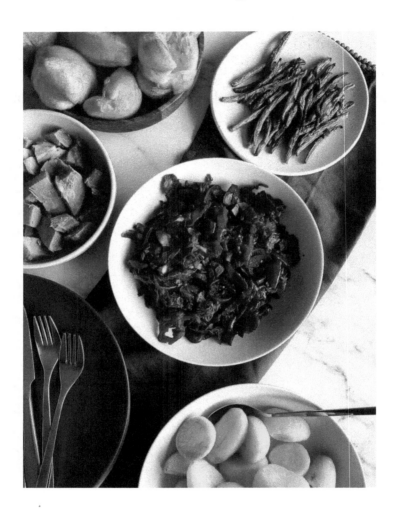

Ingredients

1 ½ pounds potatoes, peeled and cut into 1-inch chunks

½ onion, thinly sliced

¼ cup vegetable stock

1 tbsp. extra virgin olive oil

Black pepper

½ pound fresh Red cabbage, roughly chopped

Directions:

Put all of the Ingredients in a slow cooker except the last one. Top with handfuls of red cabbage and stuff the slow cooker with it. If you can't fit it all in at once, let the first batch cook first and add some more red cabbage. Cook for 3or 4 hours on medium until potatoes become soft. Scrape the sides and serve.

Endive & Kohlrabi in Pesto Sauce

Ingredients

1 ½ pounds kohlrabi, peeled and cut into 1-inch chunks

½ onion, thinly sliced

¼ cup vegetable stock

1 tbsp. extra virgin olive oil 2 tbsp. pesto sauce

Black pepper

½ pound fresh endive, roughly chopped

Directions:

Put all of the Ingredients in a slow cooker except the last one. Top with handfuls of endive and stuff the slow cooker with it. If you can't fit it all in at once, let the first batch cook first and add some more endive. Cook for 3or 4 hours on medium until kohlrabi become soft. Scrape the sides and serve.

Slow Cooked Choy Sum in Yellow Bean Sauce

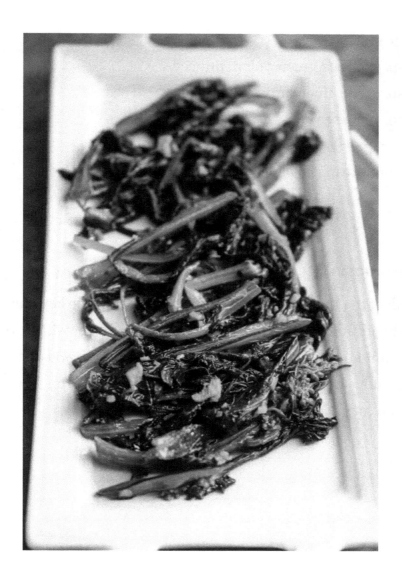

Ingredients

1 ½ pounds turnips, peeled and cut into 1-inch chunks

½ onion, thinly sliced

¼ cup vegetable stock

1 tbsp. sesame seed oil

2 tbsp. chopped green onion, minced

4 tbsp. garlic, finely minced

2 tbsp. Chinese yellow bean sauce

Black pepper

½ pound fresh choy sum, roughly chopped

Directions:

Put all of the Ingredients in a slow cooker except the last one. Top with handfuls of choy sum and stuff the slow cooker with it. If you can't fit it all in at once, let the first batch cook first and add some more choy sum. Cook for 3or 4 hours on medium until turnips become soft. Scrape the sides and serve.

Slow Cooked Watercress and Chanterelle Mushrooms

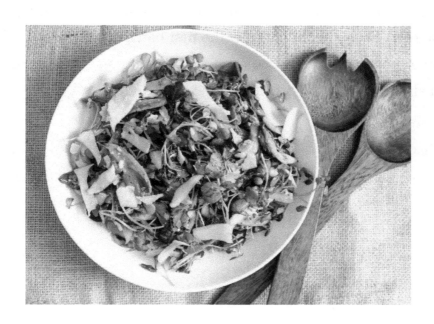

Ingredients

1 ½ pounds chanterelle mushrooms

½ onion, thinly sliced

¼ cup vegetable stock

1 tbsp. extra virgin olive oil

Rainbow peppercorns

½ pound fresh watercress, roughly chopped

Directions:

Put all of the Ingredients in a slow cooker except the last one. Top with handfuls of watercress and stuff the slow cooker with it. If you can't fit it all in at once, let the first batch cook first and add some more watercress Cook for 3or 4 hours on medium until mushrooms become soft. Scrape the sides and serve.

Slow-cooked Porcini Mushrooms and Watercress

Ingredients

1 ½ pounds porcini mushrooms

½ onion, thinly sliced

¼ cup vegetable stock

1 tbsp. canola oil

2 tbsp. minced garlic

Black pepper

½ pound fresh watercress, roughly chopped

Directions:

Put all of the Ingredients in a slow cooker except the last one. Top with handfuls of watercress and stuff the slow cooker with it. If you can't fit it all in at once, let the first batch cook first and add some more watercress. Cook for 3or 4 hours on medium until mushrooms become soft. Scrape the sides and serve.

Slow Cooked Shitake Mushroom and Spinach in Hoi sin Sauce

Ingredients

1 pound shitake mushrooms, coarsely chopped

½ onion, thinly sliced

¼ cup vegetable stock

1 tbsp. sesame oil

2 tbsp. hoi sin sauce

Black pepper

½ pound fresh spinach, roughly chopped

Directions:

Put all of the Ingredients in a slow cooker except the last one. Top with handfuls of spinach and stuff the slow cooker with it. If you can't fit it all in at once, let the first batch cook first and add some more spinach. Cook for 3or 4 hours on medium until mushrooms become soft. Scrape the sides and serve.

Slow Cooked Curried Choy Sum & Button Mushrooms

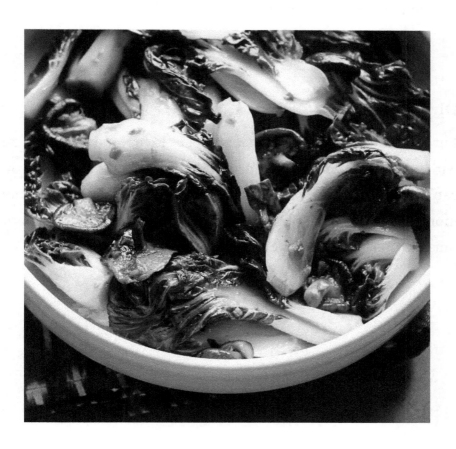

Ingredients

1 ½ pounds button mushrooms

½ onion, thinly sliced

¼ cup vegetable stock

1 tbsp. extra virgin olive oil

1 tbsp. curry powder

Black pepper

½ pound fresh choy sum, roughly chopped

Directions:

Put all of the Ingredients in a slow cooker except the last one. Top with handfuls of choy sum and stuff the slow cooker with it. If you can't fit it all in at once, let the first batch cook first and add some more choy sum. Cook for 3or 4 hours on medium until mushrooms become soft. Scrape the sides and serve.

Slow cooked Collard Greens & Portobello Mushrooms

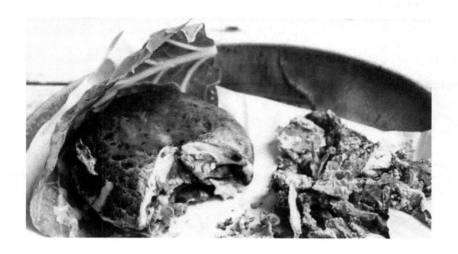

Ingredients

1 ½ pounds Portobello mushrooms

½ onion, thinly sliced

¼ cup vegetable stock

1 tbsp. extra virgin olive oil

2 tbsp. pesto sauce

Black pepper

½ pound fresh collard greens, roughly chopped

Directions:

Put all of the Ingredients in a slow cooker except the last one. Top with handfuls of collard greens and stuff the slow cooker with it. If you can't fit it all in at once, let the first batch cook first and add some more collard greens. Cook for 3or 4 hours on medium until mushrooms become soft. Scrape the sides and serve.

Slow cooked Endives and Porcini Mushrooms

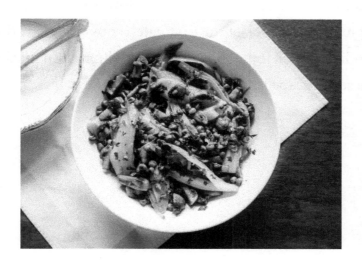

Ingredients

1 ½ pounds porcini mushrooms

½ onion, thinly sliced

¼ cup vegetable stock

1 tbsp. extra virgin olive oil

2 tbsp. pesto sauce

1 tsp. Italian seasoning

Black pepper

½ pound fresh endives, roughly chopped

Directions:

Put all of the Ingredients in a slow cooker except the last one. Top with handfuls of endives and stuff the slow cooker with it. If you can't fit it all in at once, let the first batch cook first and add some more endives. Cook for 3 or 4 hours on medium until mushrooms become soft. Scrape the sides and serve.

Slow Cooked Kale and Button Mushrooms

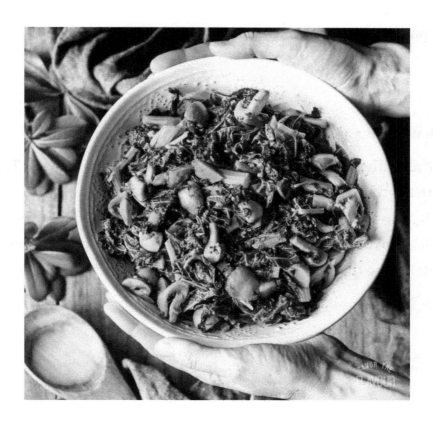

Ingredients

1 ½ pounds button mushrooms

½ onion, thinly sliced

¼ cup vegetable stock

1 tbsp. extra virgin olive oil

1 tsp. cumin

1 tsp. annatto seeds

1 tsp. olives

Black pepper

½ pound fresh Kale, roughly chopped

Directions:

Put all of the Ingredients in a slow cooker except the last one. Top with handfuls of Kale and stuff the slow cooker with it. If you can't fit it all in at once, let the first batch cook first and add some more Kale. Cook for 3or 4 hours on medium until mushrooms become soft. Scrape the sides and serve.

Slow Cooked Romaine Lettuce and Chanterelle Mushrooms

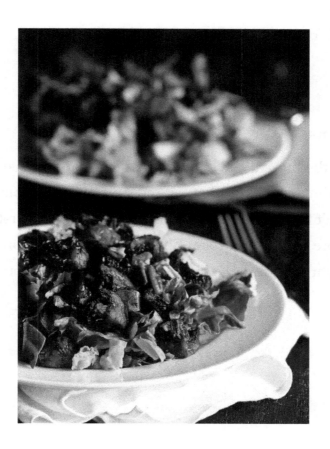

Ingredients

1 ½ pounds chanterelle mushrooms

½ onion, thinly sliced

¼ cup vegetable stock

1 tbsp. extra virgin olive oil

1 tsp. garlic powder

1 tsp. onion powder

Black pepper

½ pound fresh romaine lettuce, roughly chopped

Directions:

Put all of the Ingredients in a slow cooker except the last one. Top with handfuls of romaine lettuce and stuff the slow cooker with it. If you can't fit it all in at once, let the first batch cook first and add some more romaine lettuce. Cook for 3or 4 hours on medium until mushrooms become soft. Scrape the sides and serve.

Slow Cooked Micro Greens in Chimichurri Sauce

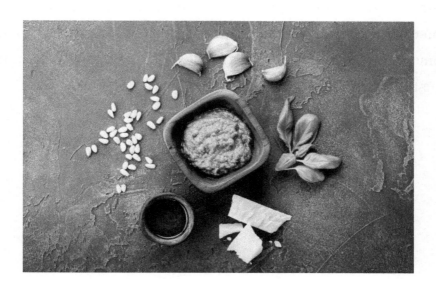

Ingredients

1 ½ pounds shitake mushrooms, sliced

½ onion, thinly sliced

¼ cup vegetable stock

1 tbsp. extra virgin olive oil

2 tbsp. chimichuri sauce

Black pepper

½ pound fresh microgreens, roughly chopped

Directions:

Put all of the Ingredients in a slow cooker except the last one. Top with handfuls of microgreens and stuff the slow cooker with it. If you can't fit it all in at once, let the first batch cook first and add some more microgreens. Cook for 3or 4 hours on medium until mushrooms become soft. Scrape the sides and serve.

Endives and Oyster Mushroom in Chimichurri Sauce

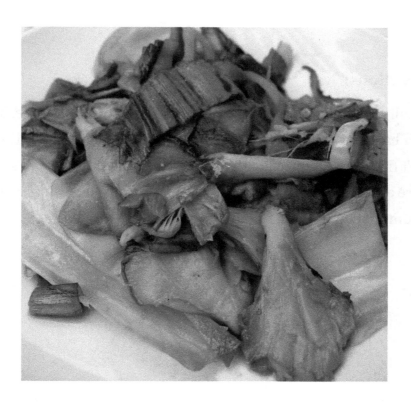

Ingredients

1 ½ pounds oyster mushrooms

½ onion, thinly sliced

¼ cup vegetable stock

2 tbsp. extra virgin olive oil

4 tbsp. chimichurri sauce

Black pepper

½ pound endives, roughly chopped

Directions:

Put all of the Ingredients in a slow cooker except the last one. Top with handfuls of endives and stuff the slow cooker with it. If you can't fit it all in at once, let the first batch cook first and add some more endives. Cook for 3or 4 hours on medium until mushrooms become soft. Scrape the sides and serve.

Triple Berry Jam

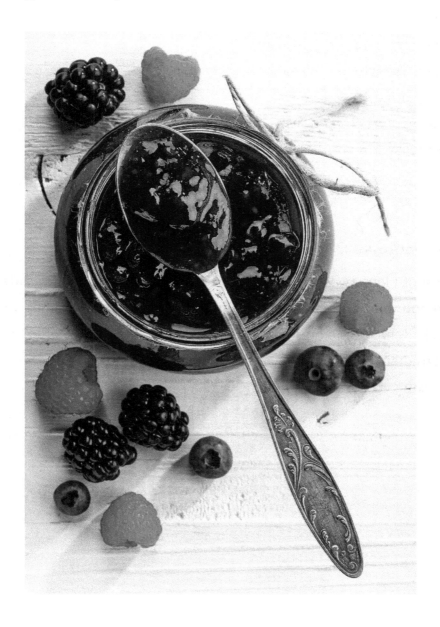

Ingredients

12 oz. blueberries, pureed

12 oz. strawberries, pureed

12 oz. raspberries, pureed

1 cup honey

2 teaspoons cinnamon

1/4 teaspoon ground ginger

Directions:

Zest of 1 lemon Cook the blueberries on low for an hour. Stir after an hour and cook for another 4 hours. Add the spices, honey and zest. Remove the lid and cook for another hour. Place all of the Ingredients in a blender and puree until smooth and store in a mason jar or container. Refrigerate.

Spicy Slow Cooked Vegetarian Tacos Main

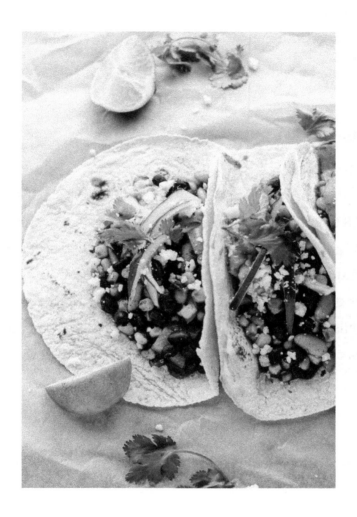

Ingredients

30 ounces red beans

1/2 cans of 15 ounces each, drained of water

1 cup corn canned, frozen or fresh

3 ounces chipotle pepper in adobo sauce, chopped

6 ounces tomato paste

1 can 3/4 cup Chili Sauce 2 tsp.

Directions:

Unsweetened Cocoa Powder 1 teaspoon Ground Cumin 1/4 teaspoon Ground Cinnamon Ingredients for Garnishing and Serving 8 taco shells hard white corn or your favorite, hard or soft favorite toppings such as lettuce, avocado, lime Sea salt Place all of the main Ingredients in a slow cooker Cook on low heat 3 1/2 hours or on high heat for 2 hours. Spread the Ingredients on the taco shells, hard or soft. Top with lettuce. Add the tomatoes, avocado, and lime. Serve with beans and rice.

Baked Chickpeas and Broccoli

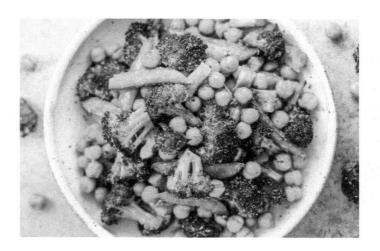

Ingredients

cooking spray

1 tablespoon olive oil

4 cloves garlic, minced

1/2 teaspoon sea salt

1/4 teaspoon ground white pepper

3 cups sliced broccoli

2 ½ cups cherry tomatoes

1 (15 ounce) can chick peas, drained

1 small lime, cut into wedges

1 tablespoon chopped fresh cilantro

Directions:

Preheat your oven to 450 degrees F. Line a baking pan with aluminum foil and grease with oil. Mix the olive oil, garlic, salt, and pepper thoroughly in a bowl. Add the broccoli, tomatoes, and garbanzo beans and combine until well coated. Spread out in the baking pan. Add the lime wedges. Bake in the oven until vegetables are caramelized, for about 25 minutes. Remove lime and top with cilantro.

Baked Carrots and Red Beets

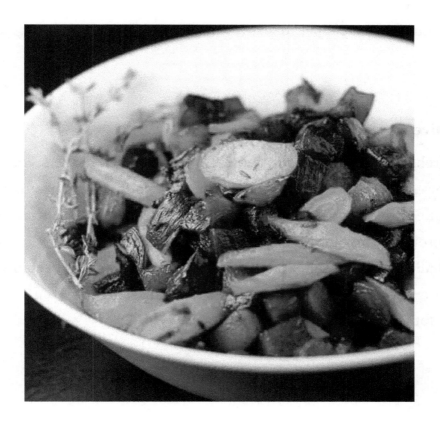

Ingredients

2 cups mini cabbages, trimmed

1 cup large Sweet potato chunks

1 cup large carrot chunks

1 cup cauliflower florets

1 cup cubed red beets

1/2 cup shallot chunks

2 tablespoons extra virgin olive oil

Sea salt

Ground Black pepper to taste

Directions:

Preheat your oven to 425 degrees F. Set the rack to the second-lowest level part of the oven. Submerge the Brussels sprouts in salted water and let it soak for 15 minutes Drain the Brussels sprouts. Combine the potatoes, carrots, cauliflower, beets, shallot, olive oil, salt, and pepper in a bowl. Layer the vegetables in a single layer onto a baking sheet. Roast in the oven until caramelized for about 45 minutes.

Baked Mini Cabbage in Balsamic Glaze

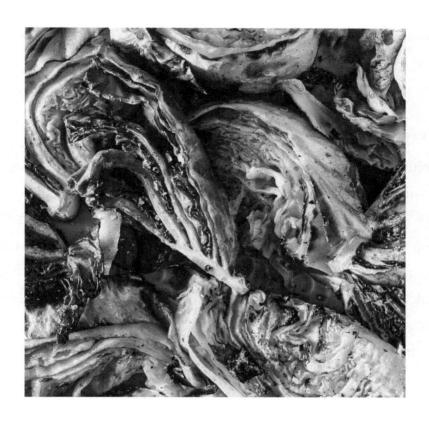

Ingredients

1 (16 ounce) package fresh mini cabbage

1 small white onion, thinly sliced

5 tablespoons olive oil, divided

1/4 teaspoon

Sea salt

1/4 teaspoon freshly Ground Black pepper

1 shallot, chopped

1/4 cup balsamic vinegar

1 teaspoon chopped dried rosemary

Directions:

Preheat your oven to 425 degrees F. Mix the mini cabbage and onion thoroughly in a bowl. Add 4 tablespoons olive oil Season with salt, and pepper Spread the cabbage on a pan. Bake in the oven until mini cabbage and onion become tender for about 28 minutes. Heat 2 tablespoons olive oil in a pan over medium-high heat. Sauté shallot until tender for about 4 minutes. Add balsamic vinegar and cook until reduced for about 5 minutes. Add the rosemary into the glaze and pour over the vegetables.

Vegetarian Taco

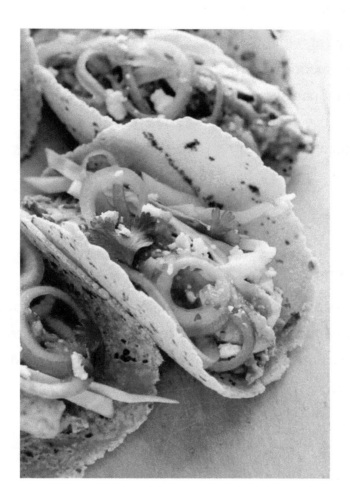

Ingredients

1 tablespoon extra virgin olive oil 1 red onion, diced

2 cloves garlic, minced

2 pcs. jalapeno, chopped

2 (14.5 ounce) cans lima beans, rinsed, drained, and mashed

2 tablespoons yellow cornmeal

Seasoning Ingredients

1 1/2 tablespoons cumin

1 teaspoon Spanish paprika

1 teaspoon cayenne pepper

1 teaspoon chili powder

1 cup salsa

Directions:

Heat olive oil over medium heat. Add the onion, garlic, and jalapeno pepper and sauté until tender. Add the mashed beans. Add the cornmeal. Add seasoning Ingredients. Cover and cook for 5 minutes.

Spicy Curried Lima Beans

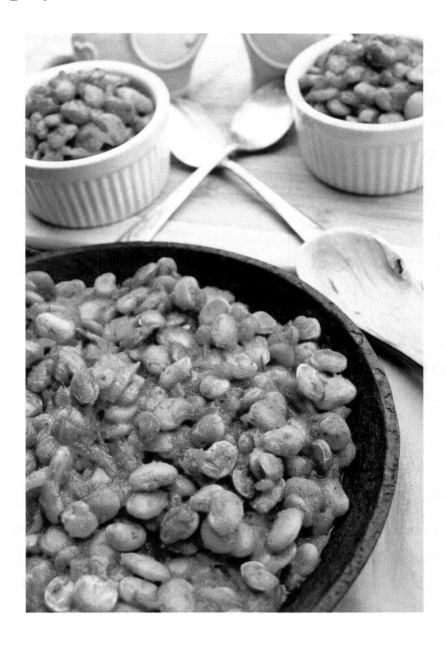

Ingredients

4 potatoes, peeled and cubed

2 tablespoons olive oil

1 yellow onion, diced

6 cloves garlic, minced

1 (14.5 ounce) can diced tomatoes

1 (15 ounce) can lima beans, rinsed and drained

1 (15 ounce) can peas, drained

1 (14 ounce) can coconut milk

Seasoning Ingredients

2 teaspoons Ground cumin

1 1/2 teaspoons cayenne pepper

1 tbsp. and 1 teaspoon curry powder

1 tbsp. and 1 teaspoon garam masala

1 (1 inch) piece fresh ginger root, peeled and minced

2 teaspoons sea salt

Directions:

Submerge the potatoes in salted water. Boil over high heat and reduce heat to medium-low. Cover and let it simmer until tender, for about 15 minutes. Drain let it dry for a minute and a half. Heat the olive oil in a skillet over medium heat. Add the onion and garlic; cook and stir until the onion turns translucent for about 5 minutes. Add the seasoning Ingredients. Cook for 2 minutes more. Stir in the tomatoes, beans, peas, and potatoes. Add the coconut milk, and simmer for 8 minutes.

Steamed Broccoli

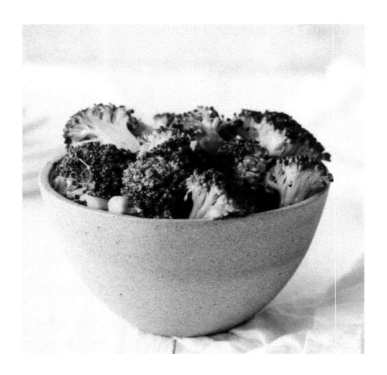

Ingredients

20 pcs. broccoli florets, preferably blanched

1 teaspoon sesame seed oil

1/4 teaspoon

Sea salt

3 cups water

Directions:

Place water in the bottom half of a steamer pan set. Add salt and oil, and bring to a boil. Place the vegetable in the top half of the steamer pan set. Steam for 5 to 10 minutes depending on the thickness of the vegetable, or until vegetable becomes tender.

Steamed Cauliflower

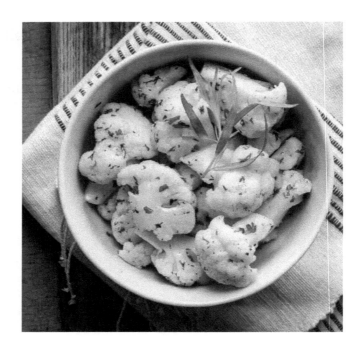

Ingredients

20 pcs. cauliflower florets, rinsed and drained

1 teaspoon canola oil

1/4 teaspoon Sea salt

3 cups water

Place water in the bottom half of a steamer pan set.

Add salt and oil, and bring to a boil.

Directions:

Place the vegetable in the top half of the steamer pan set. Steam for 5 to 10 minutes depending on the thickness of the vegetable, or until vegetable becomes tender.

Steamed Choy Sum

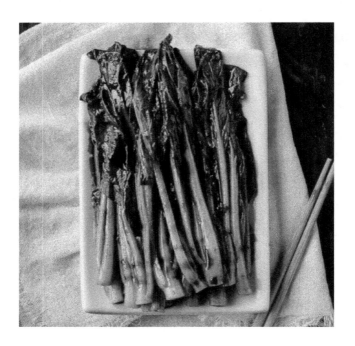

Ingredients

1 bunch choy sum

1 teaspoon sesame oil

1/4 teaspoon Sea salt

3 cups water

Place water in the bottom half of a steamer pan set.

Add salt and oil, and bring to a boil.

Directions:

Place the vegetable in the top half of the steamer pan set. Steam for 5 to 10 minutes depending on the thickness of the vegetable, or until vegetable becomes tender.

Stir Fried Sweet Potatoes

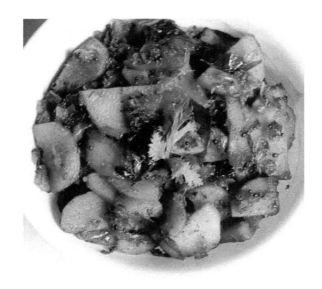

Ingredients

1 onion, chopped

1/4 cup extra virgin olive oil

1 pound sweet potatoes, peeled and cubed

1 teaspoon Sea salt Spice Mix

1/2 teaspoon cayenne pepper

1/4 teaspoon Ground turmeric

1/4 teaspoon Ground cumin

2 tomatoes, chopped

Directions:

Sauté and brown the onion in oil in a pan. Add the sea salt, cayenne, turmeric and cumin. Stir in the potatoes and cook while stirring frequently for 10 min. Stir in the tomatoes and cover Cook until potatoes become soft, for about 11 minutes.

Simple Red Bean and Jalapeno Burrito

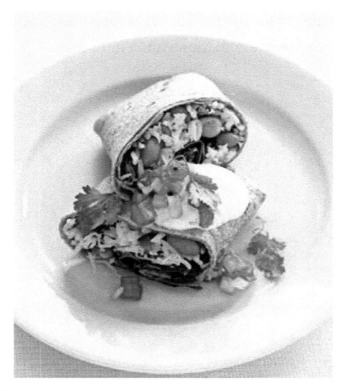

Ingredients

2 (10 inch) flour tortillas

2 tablespoons olive oil

1 small red onion, chopped

1/2 green bell pepper, chopped

2 teaspoon minced garlic

1 (15 ounce) can red beans, rinsed and drained

1 teaspoon minced jalapeno peppers

3 ounces ricotta cheese

1/2 teaspoon Sea salt

2 tablespoons chopped fresh cilantro

Wrap tortillas in a foil Bake them in a preheated 350 degree oven for 15 minutes.

Directions:

Heat oil in a pan over medium heat. Place red onion, bell pepper, garlic and jalapenos in a pan. Cook for 2 minutes while stirring occasionally. Pour the beans into the pan and cook for 3 minutes while constantly stirring. Cut dairy free cream cheese into cubes and add to the pan with salt. Cook for 2 minutes while stirring. Add cilantro into this mixture. Spoon this evenly on the center of every warmed tortilla and roll the tortillas up.

Ramen and Tofu Stir Fry with Sweet and Sour Sauce

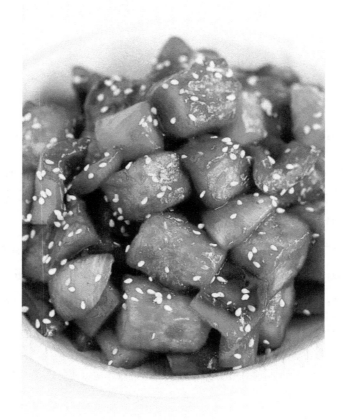

Ingredients

1 (3.5 ounce) package ramen noodles (such as Nissin(R) Top Ramen)

3 tablespoons sesame seed oil

1 slice firm tofu, cubed

1/2 thai bird chillies, chopped

1/4 small red onion, chopped

1/3 cup plum sauce

1/3 cup sweet and sour sauce

Directions:

Boil a pot of lightly salted water. Cook the noodles in boiling water and stir occasionally, until noodles are tender but still firm to the bite, 2 to 3 minutes. Drain the noodles. Heat oil in a pan over high heat. Place the tofu on one side of the pan. Place the chilies and the red onion on the other side of the pan. Cook a tofu until browned on all sides for 2 minutes. Cook and stir onion and pepper until browned, 2 minutes. Stir in the noodles into the pan Combine the noodles, tofu, onion, and pepper. Pour the plum sauce and sweet and sour sauce over the noodle. Sauté until well-combined for 3 minutes.

Spicy Curried Purple Cabbage

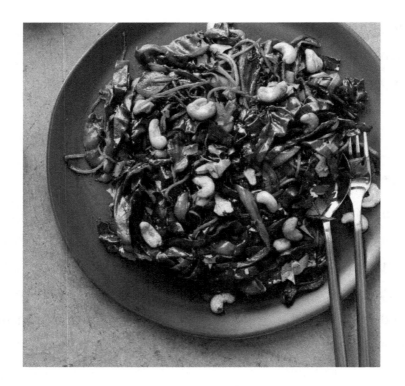

Ingredients

3 tablespoons olive oil

2 dried red chili peppers, broken into pieces

2 tsp. skinned split black lentils (urad dal)

1 teaspoon split Bengal gram (chana dal)

1 teaspoon mustard seed

1 sprig fresh curry leaves

1 pinch asafoetida powder

4 green chili peppers, minced

1 head purple cabbage, finely chopped

1/4 cup frozen peas (optional)

salt to taste

1/4 cup grated coconut

Directions:

Heat the oil in pan on medium-high heat Fry the red peppers, lentils, Bengal gram, and mustard seed in the oil. When the lentils begin to brown, add the curry leaves and asafoetida powder and stir. Add the green chili peppers and cooking for a minute more. Combine the cabbage and peas into this mixture. Season with sea salt. Cook until the cabbage wilts, for about 10 minutes. Add the coconut to the mixture and cook for 2 minutes more.

Pesto Zucchini Noodles

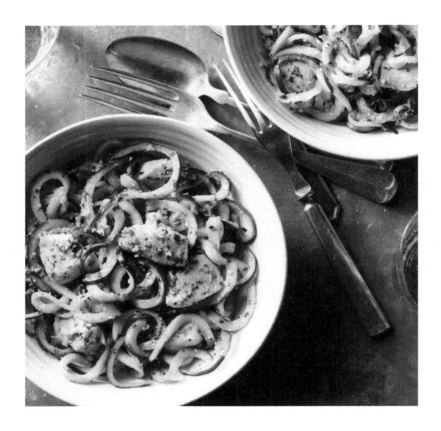

Ingredients

1 tablespoon extra virgin olive oil

4 small zucchini, cut into noodle-shape strands

1/2 cup drained and rinsed chickpeas

3 tablespoons pesto, salt and

Ground Black pepper to taste

2 tablespoons parmesan cheese

¼ cup grated gouda cheese

Directions:

Heat olive oil in a pan over medium heat Cook the zucchini until tender for around 8 minutes. Add the chickpeas and pesto to the zucchini. Lower the heat to medium-low. Cook until the chickpeas are warm and zucchini is coated for about 5 minutes Season with salt and pepper. Transfer zucchini to a bowl and top with vegan cheese.

Simple Caramelized Carrots

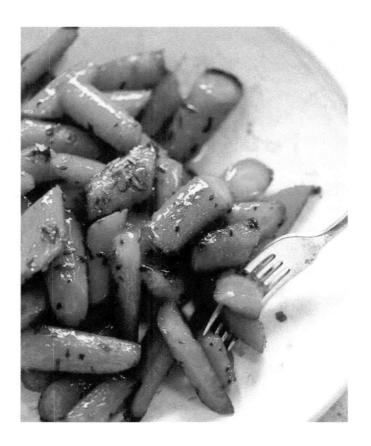

Ingredients

3 tbsp olive (a vegan brand, such as Earth Balance)

4 carrots (sliced into ¼ inch thick slices)

2 tbsp maple syrup

Directions:

Heat the olive oil on low. Add the carrots Increase the heat to medium-high and add the honey. Let the carrots cook Stir frequently until soft.

Cauliflower and Carrot Stir-fry Batter

Ingredients

1 tablespoon cornstarch

1 1/2 cloves garlic, crushed

1 teaspoon chopped fresh ginger root, divided

Ingredients

1/4 cup olive oil, divided

1 small head cauliflower, cut into florets

1/2 cup snow peas

3/4 cup julienned carrots

1/2 cup halved green beans

2 tablespoons soy sauce

2 1/2 tablespoons water

1/4 cup chopped red onion

1/2 tablespoon

Sea salt

1 teaspoons chopped fresh ginger root

Directions:

In a bowl, combine the batter Ingredients and 2 tablespoons olive oil until cornstarch dissolves. Combine the broccoli, snow peas, carrots, and green beans, tossing to lightly coat. Heat remaining 2 tablespoons oil in a pan over medium heat. Cook vegetables for 2 minutes Add the soy sauce and water. Add the onion, salt, and remaining 1 teaspoon ginger. Cook until vegetables are tender but still crisp.

Roasted Winter Squash

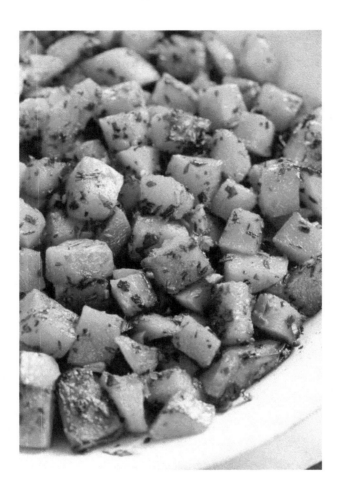

Ingredients

One 3-pound winter squash-peeled, seeded and cut into 1-inch dice

2 tablespoons extra-virgin olive oil

1 1/2 teaspoons Ground cumin

1 teaspoon Ground parsley

1/4 teaspoon cayenne pepper

Kosher salt and freshly Ground pepper

Directions:

Preheat your oven to 425°. In a bowl, combine the squash with the olive oil, cumin, coriander and cayenne. Season with salt and pepper. Layer the squash on a baking pan Roast in your oven for about 40 minutes or until tender

Baked Summer Squash and Red Bell Peppers

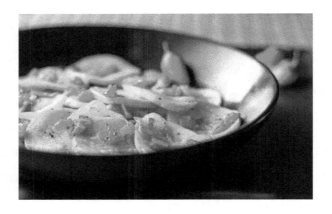

Ingredients

1 small summer squash, cubed

2 red bell peppers, seeded and diced

1 sweet potato, peeled and cubed

3 Yukon Gold potatoes, cubed

1 red onion, quartered

1 tablespoon chopped fresh thyme

2 tablespoons chopped fresh rosemary

1/4 cup extra virgin olive oil

2 tablespoons balsamic vinegar

Sea salt

Freshly Ground black pepper

Directions:

Preheat your oven to 475 degrees F. Combine the squash, red bell peppers, sweet potato, and potatoes thoroughly. Separate the red onion quarters and add them. Combine the thyme, rosemary, olive oil, vinegar, salt, and pepper. Toss this together with vegetables. Layer on a large roasting pan. Roast for 38 minutes in the oven, while stirring every 10 minutes, or until vegetables start to brown.

Vegetarian Enchilada

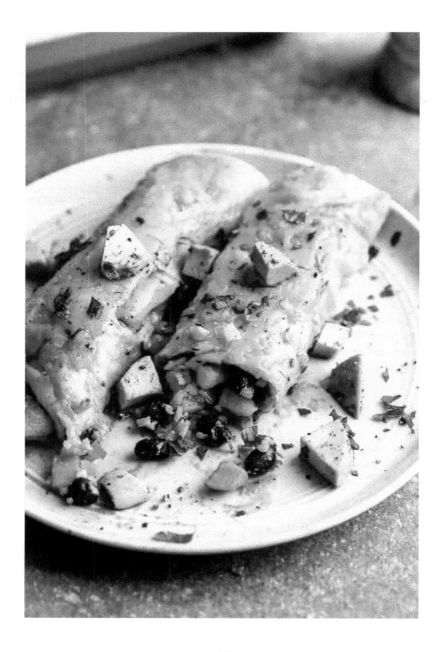

Ingredients

1 Tbsp canola oil

1 1/4 cups chopped red onion (1 medium)

1 1/4 cups chopped green bell pepper (1 medium)

5 cloves garlic, minced

1 1/2 cups dry quinoa

2 1/4 cups vegetable stock

1 (14.5 oz) can tomatoes with green chilies, not drained

1 8 oz can tomato sauce

2 tbsp. chili powder

1 1/2 tsp Ground cumin

Salt and freshly Ground black pepper, to taste

1 (14.5 oz) can black beans, drained and rinsed

1 (14.5 oz) can pinto beans, drained and rinsed

1 1/2 cups frozen corn

1 1/2 cups gouda cheese, shredded

Sea salt

Black pepper Toppings:

Diced avocados, diced Roma tomatoes, chopped cilantro, lime wedges, chopped green onions

Directions:

Heat oil in a pan over medium. In this oiled pan, sauté onion and bell pepper for 3 minutes. Add in the garlic and sauté 30 seconds longer. Pour the contents of the pan into a slow cooker. Cover and cook on high for 3 hours Add the corn and beans. Combine well and top with vegan cheese. Cover and cook until for 13 minutes longer.

Slow Cooked Macaroni and Vegan Cheese

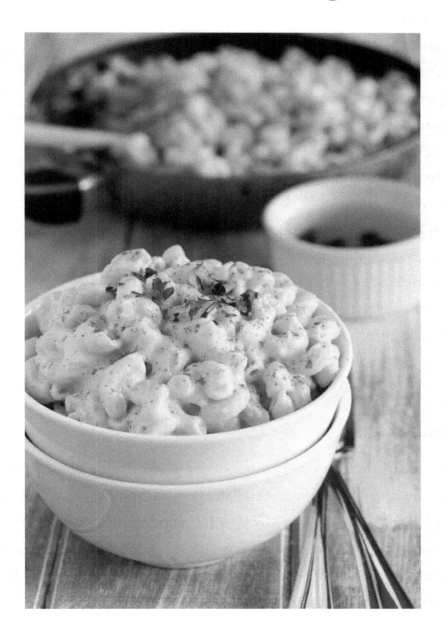

Ingredients

1 red onion, medium chopped

1 green bell pepper chopped

15 ounce can black beans rinsed and drained

15 ounce can garbanzo beans rinsed and drained

28 ounce crushed tomatoes

1 ½ tablespoons chili powder

2 teaspoons cumin

½ teaspoon salt

1/8 teaspoon Black pepper

2 cups vegetable stock

8 ounces whole wheat elbow macaroni pasta uncooked

1 ½ cups Vegan Cheese (Tofu Based)

chopped green onions for serving

Directions:

Put all of the Ingredients except for pasta, vegan cheese, and green onions in your slow cooker. Combine and cover. Cook on high heat for 4 hours or low heat for 7 hours. Add the pasta and cooking on high heat for 18 minutes, or until pasta becomes al dente Add 1 cup of cheese and stir. Garnish with the remaining vegan cheese and green onions

Fettuccini and Pesto

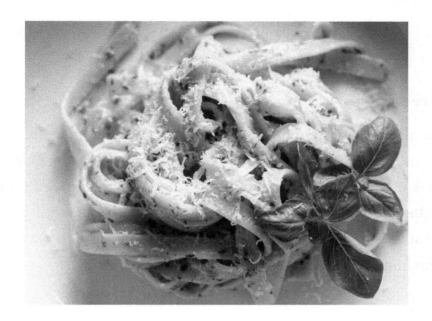

Ingredients

15 ounce can kidney beans

15 ounce can black beans

28 ounce crushed tomatoes

4 tbsp. pesto

1 tsp. Italian seasoning

½ teaspoon salt

1/8 teaspoon Black pepper

2 cups vegetable stock

8 ounces fettuccini uncooked

1 ½ cups Vegan Cheese (Tofu Based)

<u>Garnishing Ingredients:</u>

chopped green onions for serving

Directions:

Put all of the Ingredients except for pasta, vegan cheese, and garnishing Ingredients in your slow cooker. Combine and cover. Cook on high heat for 4 hours or low heat for 7 hours. Add the pasta and cooking on high heat for 18 minutes, or until pasta becomes al dente Add 1 cup of cheese and stir. Sprinkle with the remaining vegan cheese and garnishing Ingredients

Penne Pasta Cream Cheese and Olives

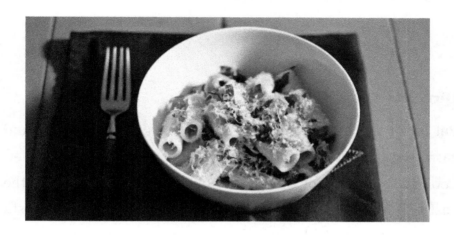

Ingredients

1 yellow onion, medium chopped

1 red bell pepper, chopped

15 ounce can butterbeans, rinsed and drained

15 ounce can garbanzo beans, rinsed and drained

28 ounce crushed tomatoes

1/4 cup green olives

2 tbsp. capers

½ teaspoon salt

1/8 teaspoon Black pepper

2 cups vegetable stock

8 ounces penne pasta uncooked

1 ½ cups Cream Cheese

<u>Garnishing Ingredients:</u>

chopped green onions for serving

Directions:

Put all of the Ingredients except for pasta, vegan cheese, and garnishing Ingredients in your slow cooker. Combine and cover. Cook on high heat for 4 hours or low heat for 7 hours. Add the pasta and cooking on high heat for 18 minutes, or until pasta becomes al dente Add 1 cup of cheese and stir. Sprinkle with the remaining vegan cheese and garnishing ingredients

Farfalle Pasta with Lima Beans and Chorizo

Ingredients

1 red onion, medium chopped

1 green bell pepper chopped

15 ounce can kidney beans

15 ounce can lima beans

28 ounce crushed tomatoes

1/4 cup vegan chorizos, coarsely chopped

1 tsp. dried thyme

½ teaspoon salt

1/8 teaspoon Black pepper

2 cups vegetable stock

8 ounces farfalle pasta uncooked

1 ½ cups Ricotta Cheese

<u>Garnishing Ingredients:</u>

chopped green onions for serving

Directions:

Put all of the ingredients except for pasta, ricotta cheese, and garnishing ingredients in your slow cooker. Combine and cover.

Cook on high heat for 4 hours or low heat for 7 hours. Add the pasta and cooking on high heat for 18 minutes, or until pasta becomes al dente Add 1 cup of cheese and stir. Sprinkle with the remaining ricotta cheese and garnishing ingredients,

Farfalle Pasta with Tomatoes and Gouda Cheese

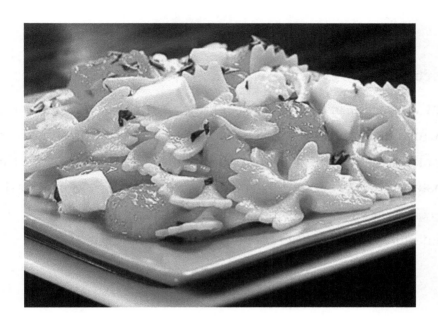

Ingredients

28 ounce crushed tomatoes

4 tbsp. pesto

1 tsp. Italian seasoning

½ teaspoon salt

1/8 teaspoon Black pepper

2 cups vegetable stock

8 ounces farfalle pasta uncooked

1 ½ cups Gouda Cheese, shredded

Garnishing Ingredients:

chopped green onions for serving

Directions:

Put all of the ingredients except for pasta, vegan cheese, and garnishing ingredients in your slow cooker. Combine and cover. Cook on high heat for 4 hours or low heat for 7 hours. Add the pasta and cooking on high heat for 18 minutes, or until pasta becomes al dente Add 1 cup of cheese and stir. Sprinkle with the remaining gouda cheese and garnishing ingredients

Penne Pasta in Spicy Chimichurri Sauce

Ingredients

1 red onion, medium chopped

1 green bell pepper chopped

15 ounce can butterbeans, rinsed and drained

15 ounce can garbanzo beans, rinsed and drained

4 tbsp. chimichurri sauce

1/2 tsp. cayenne pepper

½ teaspoon salt

1/8 teaspoon Black pepper

2 cups vegetable stock

8 ounces penne pasta uncooked

Garnishing ingredients:

chopped green onions for serving

1 ½ cups Cream Cheese

Directions:

Put all of the ingredients except for pasta and garnishing ingredients in your slow cooker. Combine and cover. Cook on high heat for 4 hours or low heat for 7 hours. Add the pasta and cooking on high heat for 18 minutes, or until pasta becomes al dente Add 1 cup of cheese and stir. Sprinkle with the remaining cream cheese and garnishing ingredients

Spaghetti with Butterbeans and Ricotta

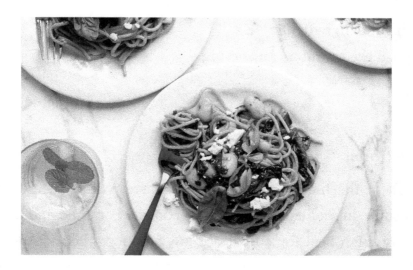

Ingredients

1 yellow onion, medium chopped

1 red bell pepper, chopped

15 ounce can butterbeans, rinsed and drained

15 ounce can black beans, rinsed and drained

28 ounce crushed tomatoes

4 tbsp. vegan cream cheese

1 tsp. herbs de Provence

½ teaspoon salt

1/8 teaspoon Black pepper

2 cups vegetable stock

8 ounces spaghetti uncooked

1 ½ cups Ricotta Cheese

Garnishing ingredients:

chopped green onions for serving

Directions:

Put all of the ingredients except for pasta, vegan cheese, and garnishing ingredients in your slow cooker. Combine and cover. Cook on high heat for 4 hours or low heat for 7 hours. Add the pasta and cooking on high heat for 18 minutes, or until pasta becomes al dente Add 1 cup of cheese and stir. Sprinkle with the remaining ricotta cheese and garnishing ingredients.

Pappardelle Pasta with Tomatoes and Garbanzo Beans

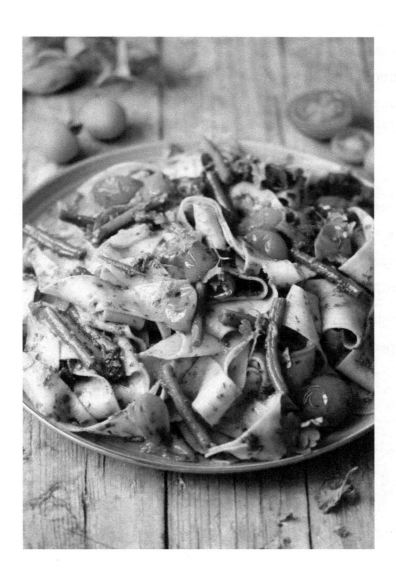

Ingredients

1 red onion, medium chopped

1 green bell pepper chopped

15 ounce can butterbeans, rinsed and drained

15 ounce can garbanzo beans, rinsed and drained

28 ounce crushed tomatoes

2 tbsp. tomato paste

1 tsp. basil

1 tsp. Italian seasoning

½ teaspoon salt

1/8 teaspoon black pepper

2 cups vegetable stock

8 ounces pappardelle pasta uncooked

1 ½ cups Vegan Cheese (Tofu Based)

Garnishing ingredients:

chopped green onions for serving

Directions:

Put all of the ingredients except for pasta, vegan cheese, and garnishing ingredients in your slow cooker. Combine and cover. Cook on high heat for 4 hours or low heat for 7 hours. Add the pasta and cooking on high heat for 18 minutes, or until pasta becomes al dente Add 1 cup of cheese and stir. Sprinkle with the remaining vegan cheese and garnishing ingredients

Lightning Source UK Ltd.
Milton Keynes UK
UKHW020659130521
383647UK00001B/90